LIFE

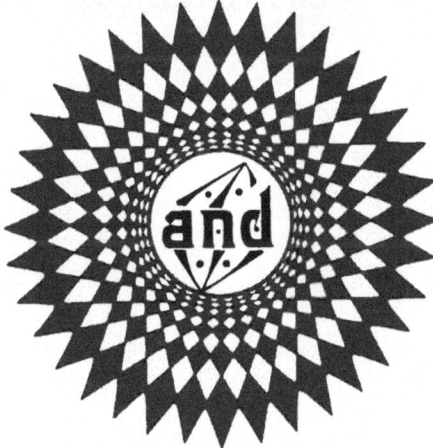

DEATH

by

George Ohsawa

George Ohsawa Macrobiotic Foundation
Chico, California

In accordance with the Bill of Rights, this publication is issued for information purposes only, is not labeling for any product, and is copyrighted under international law, which prohibits reprinting in whole or part without written permission from the George Ohsawa Macrobiotic Foundation.

First Edition   1971
Current Edition (minor edits)   2013 Dec 1

© copyright 1971 by
George Ohsawa Macrobiotic Foundation
    PO Box 3998, Chico, California 95927-3998
    530-566-9765; fax 530-566-9768
    www.ohsawamacrobiotics.com; gomf@ohsawamacrobiotics.com

Published with the help of East West Center for Macrobiotics
    www.eastwestmacrobiotics.com

ISBN 978-0-918860-03-3

Contents

Part One

Life and Death

Regarding Life and Death, Oriental and Occidental thought are completely opposite to one another, as is clearly apparent in *Life* magazine (August 6, 1965) and *Time* magazine (September 24 and November 12, 1965).

"Man dies a little each day."

And explains:

"In spite of the development of medicine, longevity has not been prolonged at all. The decrease in infant mortality creates the statistical illusion that the life span for Americans has been increased...

"The nourishment of American infants is particularly harmful...

"Knowledgeable gerontologists (specialists in problems of old age) do not believe in the existence of a drug that can prolong life...

"Science has very slowly increased longevity but has not fortified human vitality at all...

"According to statistics, if heart and kidney diseases were completely eliminated, longevity in general would be increased by no more than ten years. The disappearance of cancer would increase it by only 1.8 years...

"Autopsies performed on young G.I.s (aged 18-22 years),

who died in the Korean War, revealed many a case of un-suspected arteriosclerosis. We are forced to conclude that gerontology must begin its research in the cradle...

"It appears to be a necessity that child specialists recon-sider their views on infant nutrition...

"It is known that among animals, the one whose head is the largest in proportion to the rest of its body, lives the longest. Take the squirrel, for example. By comparison to its body, its head is the largest of all. It lives the longest. And incidentally, its intelligence is superior... *(See Edi-tor's note on page 19.)

"No one dies of old age. Everyone dies of some disease, e.g., diverse heart ailments, diabetes, rheumatism, neural-gia, cancer...

"The head—only 2% of the total body weight—consumes 25% of the oxygen assimilated by the organism...

"Each day sees the destruction of several million human body cells...

"According to gerontology, the principal cause of aging is rapid hardening of collagen or connective tissue, a kind of simple-protein that is found everywhere—beneath the skin, in the cartilage, filling intercellular space. It forms 30% of the total protein in the body. The suppleness and elasticity of babies is a direct product of new collagen...

"When collagen gets hardened, there is no hope that it will recover its flexibility. A certain Dr. Corn, however, is ex-perimenting with mice on the premise that bean protein will be helpful in combatting this condition...

"The Academy of Gerontology receives more than three million dollars in donations per year, besides which the U.S. Department of Health grants thirty times that amount for research in the same field...

"Some think it appropriate to study the future and treatment of "healthy" oldsters in our society since the cause of old age will be uncovered before long. Others (like Dr. M. C. of the Boston University Medical Faculty) think gerontological research has not gone beyond the level of cancer research, fifteen years ago..." (*Life* Magazine)

As we study material such as this from *Life*, it seems apparent that *death* is the most important discovery in the Occident over the centuries; its prime motivation. The Orient, by contrast, found *life*.

The Occident was and still is terror-stricken by its discovery. The Orient cried out in joy and passionate wonder. What an example of the front and back of the same coin.

This is why the Occident has been the birthplace of science, physics, the study of the realm of matter... all hyper-involvements with the visible world. The Orient, on the other hand, gave birth to religion, to the study of the Tao and metaphysics, to the study of spirituality and the invisible world.

Occidental medicine draws its motive power from the dead body, e.g., autopsies, microscopic study of slides prepared from fixed dead material, alleviation of suffering; the medicine of the Extreme Orient from the discovery of the grandeur of the Universe and spirituality. (See *The Yellow Emperor's Book of Internal Medicine*. Ed.)

In an article entitled, "Death is our Constant Companion," *Time* declares:

"For man, there exists no more oppressive thought than this:

"We must inevitably die...

"Civilization is a fortress whose foundation sinks deep into the world of death...

"The Egyptians made a vast cemetery and garden of soul out of their entire land...

"The spoils of war were not what motivated the Aztecs to conquer Mexico. They were spurred on by the desire to satisfy the cruel greed of the carnivorous gods...

"Man has erected vast constructions of the intelligence in order to overcome the torments and horrors of Death:

> "All philosophies from that of Socrates 2300 years ago to that of Karl Jaspers today have only been efforts at preparing man for death. Many others have endeavored to render death impotent, be it by magic or by reason...

"Death is nothing to us because what is dispersed is incapable of feeling; what cannot feel at all is nothing, according to Epicurus...

"Montaigne repeated this sentiment in his celebrated formulation:

> "Death is of no concern to us whether we are alive or dead. If we are alive, we exist and we are not troubled. If we are dead, it matters not—we exist no longer...

"The Three Fates are armed with great shears while Father Time holds a menacing scythe...

"The great effort of Christianity is to overcome death:

> "Oh death, where is thy victory?
> "Oh death, where is thy sting?
> "cried Paul the Apostle...

"The skeleton that sits astride the pale blue steed in the Apocalypse laughs hollowly..." (*Time* magazine.)

This is the sort of judgment that exerts its power over the earth;

it annoys men, pressures them, terrorizes them into both sublime and violent conduct.

In the Occident and especially the United States today, the attitude toward the mystery of death is to turn away completely from established tradition.

The medical point of view makes it appear that death has been deferred more and more. Scholars like Norbert Wiener seriously believe that we can prolong human life for as long as we care to. Yet they tremble at the thought of the time not too distant when man will have completely over-populated the earth.

Socially speaking, man has become more and more inhuman and close-fisted as regards the ceremonials of death and mourning. Only the passing of a Kennedy or a Churchill brings to our ears, once more, the sad sound of the funeral drums.

From the religious viewpoint, the assurance and even the idea of immortality have become quite obscure and inexact. The eventuality of death, once dominated by dark mystery and horror, is completely forgotten. In this, there is very deep significance.

THE RATIONALIZATION OF DEATH

In the thinking of modern man, the problem of death is left out of the questions like:

> Who are we?
> How should we live?

Man's thinking does not link his ephemeral life to those sources in mythology which are his hereditary wealth, born of hope and astonishment. Modern man uses all his power to eradicate the unhappy finality...death.

For Carl Jung, death gives life its reason for being. He is quite opposed to the abandonment of the traditional judgment that upheld this way of seeing death. He warns us that we must stop thinking of death as an end without meaning.

Psychologist Rollo May says the same thing: to consider death as a final point is to deprive life of all meaning, render it absurd and hateful.

To consider death as no more than the end result of ordinary, mechanical life—an accident of nature—is to dodge the problem.

In former days, mothers and babies often died in child birth. Today this occurs much less frequently. Men meet death face-to-face less often all the time. Pain, the doctor's visit, intimate sadness, last heart-rending farewells...all is relegated to the background. When our T.V. babies learn that grandfather has passed away, their only concern is, "From what?"

As doctors discuss the handling of death with hospital advisors, the talk focuses on one point..."How can we decrease a man's final suffering?" Would this not be the concern of the undertaker?

The second point that receives much attention is this one: should invalids be told of approaching death? Most doctors are opposed to giving a warning. But psychoanalysts are certain that doctors are very fearful of death, that they flee from the whole idea because victorious death is their most fearsome enemy...the sign of their defeat. One investigation has shown that doctors, from childhood on, have more of the fear of death than the average person. Dr. H. F. of Los Angeles has deduced that this very fear is what leads them to become doctors.

At one time people sought to avoid sudden, violent death. Today, however, there seems to be a preference for it. For example, deaths resulting from car or plane accidents, from war or crime, are sudden and violent. There is the sudden heart attack, the unexpected cerebral hemorrhage caused by hypertension. Modern death is very abrupt and leaves no time for thought of what is beyond. Before one can consider the hereafter, he is already in the comatose state.

The third question—knowing when to free a patient from the

suffering of death—is no less pressing. Whether from the human or sentimental standpoint, does one man have the right to arbitrarily end the suffering of another?

In London, Dr. C. Saunders, of St. Joseph's Hospital for incurable patients, has made an art of the psychological preparation of patients for death. All his effort is toward orienting patients to approaching death and permitting them to enjoy their last remaining days or weeks as much as possible. "This is the time when man accepts, psychologically speaking, that state which is the most natural one in his life."

SIMPLIFICATION OF MOURNING

The problem of death is treated in the same manner that sexuality was dealt with in the literature of the Victorian era.

To mourn the dead is no longer stylish. Funeral services have become more and more simple. They have become so simple and short that undertakers themselves are shocked.

According to the director of the Technical School of Interment at Dallas, Texas, the course offered there used to concentrate on the techniques of embalming. Today, four hours are devoted to that study while the rest of the time, nineteen hours to be exact, is given to other theories and techniques, the principal one of which is "How to Assume a Funeral Attitude Without Truly Being Affected By It!"

Mourning dress, the veil, the black hat, the arm band—all are passe. The unwritten law that inhibited people from remarrying immediately after the death of a loved one is a thing of the past.

Tennyson said:

"If there were no eternal life, I would throw myself into the sea!"

And Bismark:

"If there were no other life after death, life itself would be valueless. It would even be useless to arise and dress in the morning."

Freud too:

"The oldest and strongest belief of man is that one which assures him that death is only an entry into a marvelous life."

Nevertheless, death today is more like a barrier than an entry. The fear of it is responsible for many a neurosis. Christianity teaches the hope of overcoming the fear of death, all the time implying that one will never have to experience it. Modern man has become increasingly materialistic in his attitude toward death; he now calls it a "giving up."

We even hear the following:

"'Actual life and life-after-death' are ideas devoid of all sense. Suicide alone makes sense for us..."

Sartre declares that life exists only for itself and that this is its entire meaning. However, man is still left with no solution as regards the void after death!

The conclusion of *Time*:

"Death is incomprehensible. We can do no more than accept it as the inseparable companion of human life..."

THE IDEA OF LIFE AND DEATH
IN THE EXTREME ORIENT

The commonly-held viewpoint of Americans concerning death (as it has been recounted in *Time* and *Life*) is joined by another product of the same kind of thinking (*Time*, 9-24-65):

War is an eternal and unavoidable condition of life.

Here we see the limits of the common sense of America, the modern World Empire.

Modern science deceives us into believing that it is in a state of constant, infinite, day-by-day development towards totality. Actually, science is bound to the relative, material world and knows nothing of the first principles of the world of metaphysics: Peace, Justice, Life, Liberty, Memory, Spirit, Will, Judgment, Health, Happiness, Truth.... (Metaphysics is the study of the infinite, absolute world.)

Here is the limit of the judgment, the intellectuality, the thought represented by America. Occidental science totally ignores the world of spirituality, happiness, Peace—as Bergson so judiciously noted—while it has pressed to the extreme its study of materiality. It is only natural that the development of weapons of death or assassination in the West has attained heights never before imagined anywhere on earth!

The course of development of man's understanding of Life in the Extreme Orient is diametrically opposite to what has occurred in the West. Oriental man's original reaction to Life was complete astonishment. In contemplating the Universe as a whole as well as those phenomena on earth, he experienced deep wonder at what he saw: forests, mountains, rivers, flowers, insects, wind and snow, rain and tempest. He was even more amazed at Life itself. He thought, reflected, meditated, and concluded that the origin of the material world is the void.

The Occidental mind cannot easily attain this deep concept of resignation and total acceptance: It has based everything to the very end on that absolute called "matter;" it is attached to matter, it believes in matter—authority, gold, knowledge—as in tutelary gods!

The thinkers of the Extreme Orient of thousands of years past—free men—were entirely immersed in meditation on the mechanism whereby the world of void (or the infinite) produces all visible phenomena. The result of their labor was the discovery of the unitary logic of Genesis and Being. This logic spread throughout the entire world, in vulgarized form, as the five great religions of the Extreme Orient.

This metaphysics or philosophy was introduced into the realm of physics (science) by the Chinese to explain the principle and mechanism of universal transmutation. Its miraculous result was the discovery of the practical alchemy of atomic transmutation. The men of China and India knew aluminum and iron thousands of years ago; they even understood the metallurgy of alloys and steel-making.

The teachings of Lao-tse, Song-tse, and Buddha as well as the philosophy of Vedanta shed a brilliant light on the essence of the cycle of life.

Without stopping at their miraculous findings, the Extreme Orientals continued to give equal attention to both metaphysics (the spiritual world) and physics (the material world). They ended by abandoning the latter; they gave up studying physics because the infinite and absolute world was more profound and much more exciting to investigate. It made one forget everything else.

The relative world being restricted and finite, they reasoned, research concerning it had a limit, an end. If one pursued it beyond that point, one burst in upon the infinite, upon unchartered, territory where the rules of the relative world do not apply. *This has happened to modern nuclear physics.*

Occidentals have enormous difficulty understanding that the Universe is Infinite, Absolute, and Eternal. For them, the principle of relativity encompasses and surpasses all! But relativity being bounded and finite, we meet that finality wherein there is nothing more to penetrate. We come to unmistakable evidence that the "beyond" is infinite and absolute; we arrive at the despair, absurdity, discouragement, and forlornness of the life of materiality.

Incidentally, Occidental mathematicians have recently made a discovery upon which they insist:

Beyond 10^{-13}, we are the abstract; from this point on, we are in the void.

Occidental science has developed over a period of several hundred years; the last thirty—the era of nuclear science—can be considered as the final stage of that development. Its last and greatest glory is a murderous weapon that has no equal: the atomic bomb. This is the exact antipode of the five great religions that are the pathways of Life, Justice, and Happiness in the Extreme Orient.

Such are the separate destinies of the Orient and the Occident.

As a child in the Orient, I was attracted by what seemed to be the cause of all tragedy in this world...the instability of existence. When it seemed that I myself was destined to leave the world tragically at the age of eighteen, victim of incurable disease, the medicine of the Extreme Orient saved me. Since then, my study has gone in a straight line starting with that medicine: from the method of longevity, the I-King, and Yin-Yang, to Lao-tse—the pinnacle of all thinking in the East.

On the way, I found the Unique Principle or rather I made the acquaintance of a Principle that is both physical and metaphysical at one and the same time: it is neither one nor the other yet is equally applicable to both; it is the Principle of Life itself. I have continued to deepen and develop it for fifty-four years. It has been published for thirty years and available in three hundred volumes, both large and small, and in several kinds of periodicals and personal journals.

If one applies the insight of this discovery to the problem of life and death, one arrives at the following conclusion:

> The Universe is a constant, centrifugal expansion (I) moving at the unmeasurable and unthinkable speed of Infinity, the Absolute, and Eternal. This centrifugal expansion immediately produces two poles (II): Yin and Yang. These two produce all phenomena. Thus is born the finite world. Of necessity, this world has an end since by definition it is finite and limited. At this final point, finite phenomena disappear instantaneously and take on the form of Infinity and the Absolute, which are their origin. This cycle repeats itself without end. The process of infinite vicissitude, or

ephemeral, endless change in the Universe, is its true countenance: This is LIFE.

Properly speaking, there is no death in this process. Life on the earth is only a tiny phase in the changing of the Infinite. "It is merely an ephemeral existence that is an infinitesimal fraction of the Infinite Universe, as brief a period of time as 10^{-13} or 10^{-27} of a second. It is an inconceivably small point that possesses neither dimension, weight, nor quantity. Rare is the individual who understands that infinite depth exists in so minute a point!"

In its mechanistic way, Occidental science too has observed an infinitesimal spatio-temporal point but has failed to see infinite profundity in it. This is a fundamental error, and it was made at the very outset. To have considered C. G. S. (centimeter, gram, second)—a relative formulation—as a universal and absolute measurement reference, to assume it to be the minimal unity of time and space, was a grave mistake. It was only an imaginary unity, a product of the relative world and thus useless in the absolute, infinite realm.

The origin of this imperfection dates back more than two thousand years to the time of the Greeks. It was perpetuated later in the work of Descartes, the French philosopher-mathematician who divided the world into "visible" and "invisible" or physical and metaphysical. Unfortunately, he forgot the invisible and explored only the visible.

Now that research in this visible world has gone about as far as it can, we must return to the original point of departure and begin metaphysical investigation anew. Prize physicist W. Heitler has pleaded for this in his *Man and Science*. After that will come the effort to unify the two—physical and metaphysical—an effort that could take several thousand years of work. If, however, the Unique Principle were introduced into Occidental civilization, science, and technique right now, these years might be saved. There seems to be no other road, no path that is shorter.

Imagine that life is a written exercise—a poem, novel, or thesis.

Punctuation outlines the space between its parts and emphasizes the points from which new episodes in the story unfold in relation to what has come before. This is why punctuation is a joy to the individual who would know the concept and totality of the writing; it forms the framework of new development. People who become attached to the words themselves and remain fixed at that level find, however, that the punctuation appears to cause either a rupture or a complete stoppage of the movement of what has been written.

The author knows his ending from the very start; wise readers must anticipate this ending and for them, the punctuation is a relaxation, a joyous pause.

To use another analogy, consider that life is a long story, say *Gone With The Wind*. Certain words and phrases keep recurring naturally. Punctuation, line spacing, open areas, and white space at the end of sentences and chapters are like the dropping of a theatre curtain or an entr'acte that allows for the preparation of new scenes in the story.

If there were no pauses, entr'actes, or open spaces, all the events in the story would be an agglutinous, paste-like mass. If we were to make such a mixture of hundreds of thousands of words, if one wrote *Gone With The Wind* without punctuation or space between the letters and words, the result would be a large complicated mess, bereft of all sense.

In the same way, if we were to print all the notes in Beethoven's Ninth Symphony with no spaces in between or if we produced all the sounds at the same time, the result would be no more than a loud noise.

If we were to project all of a movie film in one second by accelerating its speed, the adventurous life of Lawrence of Arabia, for instance, would resemble a wildly abstract painting.

If all the atoms that make up your loved one were condensed so that there would be no empty space at all between the nuclei and electrons of which she is made, you would be left holding a pinpoint that weighed 40-45 kilograms. How would you ever find her kissable face and eyes?

Man falls in love, hates, cries, kills; the sum total of his activity exists thanks to space and the illusions that populate it.

In the Extreme Orient, life and its phenomena—a world of illusion—were thought to be beautiful but ephemeral like a bubble, a rose-colored mist that evaporates in the heat of the sun, a floating world of pathetic fragility. One loved it and yearned for it as one yearns for a treasure that appears only in a dream.

After a delay of several thousand years, Occidentals have at last discovered that matter is "a mathematical singularity haunting space." (*Matter*, (Lapp) Life Science Library.) But those years of thinking of matter as the final point of all things have left Occidentals at a disadvantage. Matter has for so long a time been their fortune and most precious treasure that, although they have at last discovered the great truth mentioned by Professor Lapp, its full significance eludes them. Furthermore, they are seriously upset by it... and with good reason.

If our world is so incomprehensible a mystery, truly a place of "Mathematical singularities," then what the West has taken for granted—the substantiality of matter—is in Oriental terms but an illusion, a bubble, an absurdity. And war, treachery, evil, assassinations, and "all of science itself" are the greatest absurdities of all. This certainly is an upsetting thought. It cannot possibly be true.

Occidentals seem to be waiting to be saved by a miracle after the ship they are on has struck an iceberg in the dark of night. "Scientific Civilization" and its shipwrecked passengers desperately seek the old road of hope, faith, charity, and superstition, which can take them back only to one place: the realization that the world of matter is but an illusion.

When the Greek, Democritus, divided the Universe into two

parts—atoms and space—he gave dualism its first impetus. When he became addicted solely to the study of atoms, space was forgotten and science was born.

Occidental science, physics, the natural science (formerly called natural philosophy) have produced scientific civilization. It developed over a period of 2500 years from Democritus' demi-dualism, the same dualism the Orient pretended to accept as if it were the real thing—monism.

Scientific civilization is just like an infant deformed by thalidomide: the illegitimate child born of a fabulous superstition. It is the offspring of an error that consists in believing that we might grasp and define life, space, and the infinite universe by the false monism of matter, in reality a blind-alley variety of dualism.

It is strange that in the Occident there have been eyes that have only seen physics; myopic eyes for which "the invisible does not exist;" eyes that accept spiritual blindness as being normal; eyes that do not see their own blindness in a metaphysical world.

Even though Occidental science (in essence only physics) was accepted in the Extreme Orient at the time of its introduction as being on the same level and of the same quality (if not a superior one) as the metaphysics taught for milleniums by the sages of the East, there remained those Oriental thinkers, nevertheless, who had eyes only for the metaphysical world.

* EDITOR'S NOTE (from page 6)

On the basis of your understanding of Yin and Yang, answer the following questions put by Mr. Ohsawa:

1. Why are the statements about the squirrel true?

2. What is the rule that governs the size of the human head?

Part Two

Life and Death

The incredible frivolity that consists in believing that one could understand infinite space by investigating only atoms has reached its glorious end in nuclear physics. It has thrust mankind to the verge of collective suicide. Those who cannot grasp this panoramic view of the impasse that faces man today cannot achieve the miracle of establishing World Peace by transmuting nuclear war.

Practical evidence of the great error of demi-dualism is easily found:

> Let us consider the hexagon. Geometrically speaking, it is produced by a combination of straight lines of the same length. "Seen through the eyes of physics," it is a figure formed by the combination of six straight lines of equal length. There are thousands of scientific definitions of the same variety:
>
>> a grain of rice is made up of 16 kinds of atoms
>>
>> man is made up of 800 billion cells
>>
>> the state consists of several parts—sovereignty, territory, and people
>>
>> the enzyme is a protein
>>
>> gravity is the force of attraction

entropy increases gradually until the universe ends and the world disappears into eternal death

the speed of light is ultimate and constant

the living being evolves from the inferior to the superior level

the secret of heredity is to be found in the gene, etc., etc....

This is like following a game of chess without ever acknowledging that the pieces do not move by themselves—that they depend upon the players to move them! Such a mechanistic viewpoint overlooks the life force completely.

A hexagon is only a minute portion of space, framed by six lines. These very lines to which we give length and position have no existence without infinite space. They could not even be born without it since length and position are born only of the mother-matrix called "space." The statement, "Six lines produce a hexagon," is as much a mistake as saying, "Six children have given birth to their mother."

Indeed, when one is called "father" or "mother" after the birth of a child, the name only serves to confirm an actuality. Parents, in reality, are no more than possible bearers of the names "father" and "mother." Their children are entirely children of infinite space, "the mother- matrix." It is infinite space, which is truly the prime origin of the "will to creation." Nothing occurs without it.

It is this infinite space that in the Extreme Orient is called "Absolute Void, Heavenly Void, Ko-Kuu, Eternity, Absolute, One, Brahman, Atama, God..." Some, like Schopenhauer and Spinoza, have perceived it; they have not grasped the fact, however, that it is the absolute void or spirituality or will that is the mother of all relative, finite existence; that the Void is absolute Authority, the Unique Order, just and sacred even unto the ultimate relative manifestation.

Schopenhauer baptized it "blind will!"

Professor Heitler, celebrated nuclear physicist, proclaims that science has outstripped its limits, that it is too adventurous in a labyrinth it cannot explore, that its situation is one of frantic folly. The only way out is a return to metaphysics.

Heitler risks the peace of his later years, the peace we all seek after the age of sixty. He braves possible persecution by sectarian scholars and thus puts us under an obligation as students of the Philosophy of the Extreme Orient. We must reflect deeply. The same is true for Professor Louis Kervran, an important figure in French physiology and biochemistry. His discovery of the effects of "Biological Transmutation; Natural Transmutation and Transmutation Under Low Energy" will bring him, in the near future, a glory in chemistry greater than that of Lavoisier.

Both Heitler and Kervran have recognized the importance of the metaphysics of the Extreme Orient. These two scholars have bestowed on me the honor of editing and writing prefaces for their works (the first in Japanese, the second in French). And I am only a foreigner without title or distinction! Their modesty, sense of Justice, and unselfishness is the ideal image of the Extreme Orient.

Alexis Carrel, Kervran and *Heitler* are the greatest thinkers that I have encountered in the Occident in fifty-three years. These three men of science have broken away from physics by moving beyond science into the realm of metaphysics and philosophy. They are the first emigres from Occidental civilization.

Nothing would please me more than to open for them infinite space, the void, the absolute world that crosses and encompasses both the metaphysical and physical realms; to firmly convince them of the infinite and eternal Order of the Universe that is freely and perpetually apparent everywhere.

By introducing this Order of the Universe to science, they might pass through the great door to the world of infinite liberty where reigns the World Peace for which humanity patiently waits.

The violation of metaphysics, matrix of physics, by the science of nature, is the tragedy of Oedipus murdering his father and violating his mother.

Oedipus put out his own eyes. And Prometheus, who had transgressed against the laws of heaven by stealing fire in order to give it to mankind, was condemned to be the living food of fierce eagles because of his crime. Even at that, it was not possible for him to atone for what he had done.

Such is the actual situation, grimly tragic, of the world today. Oedipus or science presses all of humanity toward a tragedy that will be the total end of scientific civilization.

Do you believe that this is humanity's fatal misadventure? I am going to analyze the situation and show you, theoretically, that such is not the case.

Changing events or "karma" are an obstacle; they are the chains that bind a slave. "An obstacle to potential exists only to be overcome." (This statement was made by Madame Bouquet, Professor at the Sorbonne and a student of the Philosophy of the Extreme Orient, at our Summer Camp in France.) The vicissitudes of life or "karma" are only an imaginary obstacle; they make man free by giving him the incentive to learn to overcome them. How grateful he must be.

In the Occident, escape by criminals and prisoners of war is an everyday occurrence, is it not?

> Liberty can be found only at the very depth of unhappiness and slavery. In a free world, liberty is not worth even one cent. Only in danger does security exist. If there were no difficulty, there would only be ease, which is monotonous. It is in the world of difficulty that we find gratitude...

It is regrettable that most so-called free men (I might even say all free men) destroy themselves for the sake of their freedom after having achieved only the first stage of it: Galileo, Giordano, Bruno, Pasteur, Lenin, Gandhi. There is no lack of related examples: Okakura, Lafcadio Hem, Itsue, Takamura, Lawrence of Arabia, Erasmus de Perse...

Those who know the Unique Principle of Macrobiotics, by contrast, never run the risk of coming to a tragic end no matter what the circumstances.

If there were no death, stories about heroic lives could not exist. If there were no space or intervals, all music including that of Bach, Beethoven, Chopin, and Wagner would not be. All arts, techniques, and actions are painted on the infinite canvas called "space." Death does not exist on this movie screen, in this time span, this void that is the great creation of infinity. Space, therefore, is not death. Infinite space, the infinite itself, is the mother-matrix of liberty. Space, the infinite void, and eternity are one.

When we will have understood that this empty space is full of an inexhaustible abundance, that it is our origin, the origin of creation and life itself, we will have come to know ourselves, to know that *we* are Life, Liberty, Omnipresence, and Omnipotence. And we will be able to prove it!

Man is free; he can do what he wills. By expending millions of dollars per day, he can kill fifty or a hundred poor women and barefooted children working in the rice fields. And to accomplish this, he can kill several hundred youngsters from his own country every week, compatriots kidnapped from their mothers. (The second World War alone caused seventy-five million young fathers or brothers to disappear.) Each day, several tens of thousands are wiped out in the name of medicine and hygiene. Education kills the judgment, instinct and intuition of millions of youths each year. Politics is a demon that absorbs the blood of three billion men.

Man is free—he can commit whatever crime he chooses. Three and one-half billion men who are not creative exercise this freedom every day. They are all criminals, all prisoners of life. For those bereft of creativity, daily life is destructive, wasteful, suicidal, deadly, in short, criminal.

Even those who are prisoners of life are expressing the Order of the Universe. Their expression of life does not recognize or take advantage of their freedom.

If one wants to take advantage of that freedom in order to enjoy the pleasure of painting beautiful pictures of flowers and butterflies or his own portrait or that of his loved one on the canvas called "space or infinite void," he has only to utilize the greatness of the grand order in infinite space. With but one person of this sort in the world, we might arrive at peace. Whoever so wishes has the opportunity to become this unique individual. All would be grateful for infinite liberty; all would be free.

The world is the scene of a Grand Theatre. We have a choice of roles: benefactor, malefactor, killer, victim, or suicide. The majority are suicides...principally the religious ones, the scholars and particularly the doctors and hygienists—killers or suicides, all. Just consider the Chief of the Center for Cancer Research...he himself was a cancer victim!

Those who do not have eternal happiness, infinite liberty, and absolute justice are killers and suicides, without exception. By comparison to these people, who are unaware of their criminality, the hit-and-run driver who hides after running down a single person is a benefactor because he *knows* his crime.

Man is free; he is infinite liberty itself. He therefore has only to do what he wishes. No one is excluded.

A life is so short that even doing what one wishes to the very utmost is still no great thing. Consider the music of Beethoven and Wagner, the work of Goethe and that of Shakespeare, the logic of Hegel, the scientific theories of Newton and Einstein, the philosophy of Kant and Descartes, the paintings of Delacroix and Picasso... are they other than mountains of paper and cloth stained with ink or color?

If you want to become an artist, thinker, or scientist like the men

I have mentioned, be the worst student of the school of Yin-Yang and the Unique Principle. And if you want to be a killer—educator, doctor, politician, promoter or industrialist—denounce the school of Yin-Yang, burn it, violate it, stone it.

You can, however, live an amusing and beautiful life in a state of poverty and obscurity; you can live a splendid independent existence without fame: merely apply Yin and Yang in your daily affairs and particularly at the table in your eating.

Whatever his path, whether he is first or last in the final analysis, man will reveal in his life the grandeur of Universal Infinite Space (Liberty), a life in which he will amuse himself with this liberty as his own possession (happiness). He can know the amusement of resolving all problems by receiving infinite energy from the prime source itself, *The Order of Infinity—Yin and Yang.*

I do not demand that you follow a certain road; the freedom of choice is yours. I only offer a guide, a map of this Life of the Universe and Infinity. I simply say this:

> Death is neither a final point nor is it the entry into the next world. Death is in reality an interval (space) at the end of the propositions and sentences of the living story of the Great Eternal Life. This interval is only a tiny gap in an infinitesimally small corner of the grand canvas of empty, infinite space. Without this canvas no world could exist. Infinite space, the Absolute, Eternity... the infinite powerplant that perpetually furnishes the energy to kindle the fires of Life.

> We must abandon the exclusivity that has brought us to the point of thinking that "our life" is ours and by us. We must recall occasionally that the great, infinite generator is our true life, the origin of our will and spirituality.

Death as the Occident has imagined it does not exist. Death resembles a camera shutter that operates 16 to 32 times per second during the course of a film, creating several million images. By repeatedly closing off the images that reach our eyes, it is the very mechanism that enables us to see movement and change. So in reality, we look at a rapid succession of fixed images. The darkness that we call death—the interruption of light—is really the mother-matrix of that light. Thus is it that in light, darkness is found...

POSTSCRIPT

No matter which images I use, they neither satisfy me nor provide a good explanation of what I am trying to convey. Yet, I must illuminate the problem of life and death for the entire world. I hope that you will give me your criticisms, questions, and ideas in regard to my thoughts. They will be very useful to me in improving my clumsy way of expressing myself.

The following additional reflections on life and death are provocative:

1. Sleep is a necessity that we cannot do without...the pursuit of activity in life is vitally dependent upon it. During sleep, all creativity, action, and thought are suspended. This same description seems to fit death also. Apparently, we are justified in saying that every time we sleep, we taste a bit of death! Sleep, then, is a little different from what we usually consider it to be. By the same token, might not death be other than what we have fearfully imagined it to be?

2. He who does not live each day in an interesting, happy, splendid, and amusing way, he who does not know the joy of living, he who moves about but is still asleep, does not understand, cannot and does not see the mechanism of the Universe. He is never awake; he is one of the living dead. Those who are unhappy in life and who end their lives full of tragic regret are slaves—people who are not wide awake,

beast-like men, the living dead...they are asleep.

3. In the course of my many trips to faraway, strange places, I have often taken warm baths. To me, the Occidental bathtub has long resembled a large coffin. Each time I relax in one, I amuse myself by imagining the day when I will be interred, stretched out, in a coffin of similar shape.

Do Occidentals also imagine—each time they take a bath—the joyous hope of the day when they will sleep their eternal sleep entirely relaxed and stretched out in that coffin? The long awaited holiday after fifty or eighty years of life—whether it has been splendid or not, happy or full of suffering. In the tub, one is completely nude, without clothes or fancy watch, stripped of power and position! What perfect carefreeness! And how much more delightful is this comfort after a hard day's work. Do Occidentals, too, think about the absurd things in the world? Don't they, too, play during this interlude at the end of the day? Don't they think, from time to time, of the day when they will be in the same position but in a coffin, when they will stretch out to their full length in that celestial bathtub?

Those who have experienced it for several hundred years should by now have enough proof of the delights of this coffin-bathtub to be full of gratitude and joy. If not, they do not deserve any more than the use of a birdbath!

4. Nowadays one can find Japanese baths throughout the Orient and particularly in Germany. They resemble the square box-like Japanese coffins of old. In this square tub, even more primitive than the tub-coffin of the West, you are forced to assume the fetal

position. This is why if you stay there quietly you are happy; you can feel the energy of the baby that is about to be born. Here we encounter again the difference between the Orient and the Occident...not only in their concept of life but in something so simple and practical as the form of the bathtub they use. It is the difference between birthplace and coffin, between life and death.

5. The relationship between death and life is comparable to the one between sleep each night and awakening each morning. Death, however, is the perfect sleep without dreams (either the ones we forget or nightmares).

Those who have these insignificant or illusionary dreams are the people whose lives are unhappy and insignificant; they are not free. Those who have horrible nightmares are exclusive, egoistic, arrogant killers. They are malefactors who violate the Order of the Universe all day long, consciously or not. If they are not already unhappy individuals every moment of their lives, they meet up with unhappiness sooner or later. Those who have trifling dreams or nightmares, those who lead an unhappy, meaningless life without liberty, begin again a similar life after death in their reincarnation. Those who lead an amusing, splendid, grateful life in the actual world have never dreamt in their previous life; that is, they have fulfilled number three of the Seven Conditions of Health:

No dreams, no movement, deep sleep.

To have a splendid life in the next world, all that is necessary is to perfect the "Seven Conditions of Health" described fully in *Macrobiotics: An Invitation to Health and Happiness*. I affirm and guarantee this on the basis of a living example: the millions of people that I have seen during fifty-three years of teaching. He who understands and fulfills the "Seven Conditions of Health" can function in a splendid, amusing, and grateful manner in this life, from here on, without waiting for the next world. Countless numbers of people have put this to the test immediately after having heard my lectures or read my books. Tens of thousands of them have understood and changed themselves rapidly and completely.

Be that as it may, those who control their dreams and achieve calm and deep sleep through Macrobiotics can be masters of their own destinies and their lives in the next world. That is why we are justified in saying that a happy or unhappy life is merely a repetition of the preceding life. (In this sense only is it justified.) I guarantee the immediate realization of a happy life in this world. I guarantee longevity as well—physiologically and biologically—through Macrobiotics.

In the fifty-three years that I have worked to spread the word of Macrobiotics, I have had an extremely amusing and adventurous life. Macrobiotics—the guarantee that everyone can lead a happy, grateful life in this world no matter where or when, and above all, from now on without waiting for the next life. I will continue on to the next scene in my joyous adventure—it is a diversion that one cannot give up even after having begun it anew a thousand times.

The fundamental religions—Buddhism, Taoism, Confucianism, Christianity—have prescribed that we do good, cultivate virtue, be honest, and refrain from killing, stealing, and committing adultery to assure ourselves happiness in the next life.

Unfortunately, we are forced to declare that this is ineffective and irrational. Above all it is utilitarian. It makes a slave of man.

Why "irrational"?

Because its mechanism cannot be explained.

Why "ineffectual"?

Because everyone carries on a bit of "black market" activity behind the scenes while on the surface apparently, he is following all the rules. And what of the people who follow all the rules blindly and hopefully yet end in unhappiness? The proof is in the large number of people who find themselves sick or unhappy after a lifetime of deep devotion to a religious discipline.

Why "utilitarian"?

This has no need of being explained because fundamentally it concerns the idea of barter.

Utilitarianism is a way of fishing for happiness in the next life with the happiness of this actual life as bait. It can be compared to a lottery in which you can not only lose your last cent, but the pitifully small, insignificant happiness of this actual world as well.

My method of absolute Macrobiotic health is just the opposite. In this case one fishes for shrimp with a whale for bait! It is endless sport telling people about Macrobiotics—the discreet key that changes reincarnation and universal metamorphosis (which some imagine is like dying in a fiery furnace) into a flying carpet.

It is like a pinball machine without a glass cover where you can move the balls at will. Each ball is a life and on this earth there are three and one half billion of them. Since our goal is to put the ball in the pocket called "happiness," everyone willingly and gladly joins in the game.

But evidently the owner of the pinball machine and his employees (aggressors called "government," capitalists, their employees, functionaries, educators, doctors, etc.) are upset by our objective. They await us in the dead of night on the road, in the doorways of our homes...they attack with all their might and attempt to throw us off the track...

This surrounding atmosphere makes our lives an adventure that is all the more lively. We never end tragically like most of the great protagonists in history and fiction—the so-called free man, the revolutionaries—because Macrobiotics is a modest method through which one wins even though vanquished and in flight: victory without arms.

As long as we continue to depend upon the kind of judgment that has taken several thousand years to discover that atoms are "finite," that declares contradictorily that "the infinite space of the Universe is limited" without having recognized that space is infinite, we are unable to understand this method of absolute health—Macrobiotics, the method for reaching supreme judgment. This is why the candidates for our School of the Unique Principle are not numerous; why most of them are utilitarians, imitators, slaves...

THE FREEDOM OF CHOICE IS OURS...

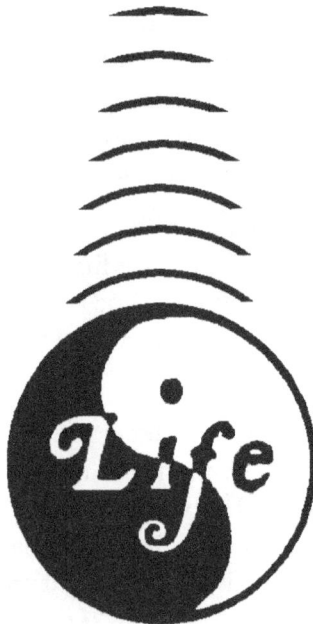

Other Books from the
George Ohsawa Macrobiotic Foundation

Acid Alkaline Companion - Carl Ferré; 2009; 121 pp.

Acid and Alkaline - Herman Aihara; 1986; 121 pp.

Basic Macrobiotic Cooking, 20th Anniversary Edition - Julia Ferré; 2007; 275 pp.

Book of Judo - George Ohsawa; 1990; 150 pp.

Cancer and the Philosophy of the Far East - George Ohsawa; 1981; 165 pp.

Essential Guide to Macrobiotics - Carl Ferré; 2011; 131 pp.

Essential Ohsawa - George Ohsawa, edited by Carl Ferré; 1994; 238 pp.

Food and Intuition 101 Volume 1: Awakening Intuition - Julia Ferré; 2012; 225 pp.

Food and Intuition 101 Volume 2: Developing Intuition - Julia Ferré; 2013; 241 pp.

French Meadows Cookbook - Julia Ferré; 2008; 275 pp.

Macrobiotics: An Invitation to Health and Happiness - George Ohsawa; 1971; 128 pp.

Philosophy of Oriental Medicine - George Ohsawa; 1991; 153 pp.

Practical Guide to Far Eastern Macrobiotic Medicine - George Ohsawa; 2010; 279 pp.

Zen Cookery - G.O.M.F.; 1985; 140 pp.

Zen Macrobiotics, Fifth Edition - George Ohsawa, edited by Carl Ferré; 2013; 219 pp.

A wide selection of macrobiotic books is available from the George Ohsawa Macrobiotic Foundation, P.O. Box 3998, Chico, CA 95965; 530-566-9765. Order toll free: 800-232-2372. Or, you may visit *www.OhsawaMacrobiotics.com* for all books and PDF downloads of many books.

www.ingramcontent.com/pod-product-compliance
Lightning Source LLC
Chambersburg PA
CBHW021343290326
41933CB00037B/719